My Stupid Cancer Journal

Cancer is my trigger. Thinking about cancer, writing about cancer, talking about cancer makes me swear like a sailor on a drunken holiday. I have now had so many situations in life connected to cancer that have made me shake uncontrollably while sobbing that I think a worldwide exception needs to be made for telling cancer to f*ck off.

[Excerpt from *Go Home Cancer, You're Drunk*]

Cover by Jessica Jack

Print: ISBN: 978-1-7373308-2-0

Printed in The United States Of America

Website: www.jessica–jack.com

IT'S ALL ABOUT ME

NAME:
PHONE:
ADDRESS:

EMERGENCY CONTACT:

ALLERGIES:

DAILY MEDICATIONS

IF LOST OR STOLEN, FOR THE LOVE OF GOD RETURN TO
THE ABOVE PERSON, THEY HAVE FREAKING CANCER AND
DO NOT NEED ANOTHER CRISIS TO DEAL WITH.

IT'S ALL ABOUT ME

DATE OF DIAGNOSIS

DIAGNOSIS

ALL THE STUPID DIAGNOSIS DETAILS

IT'S ALL ABOUT ME

IF YOUR CANCER IS A COMPLICATED BONEHEAD, AND
HONESTLY, MOST ARE...YOU MAY NEED A SECOND PAGE.
IF NOT THIS IS A GREAT PLACE TO JOT DOWN NETFLIX
SHOWS YOU WANT TO BINGE.

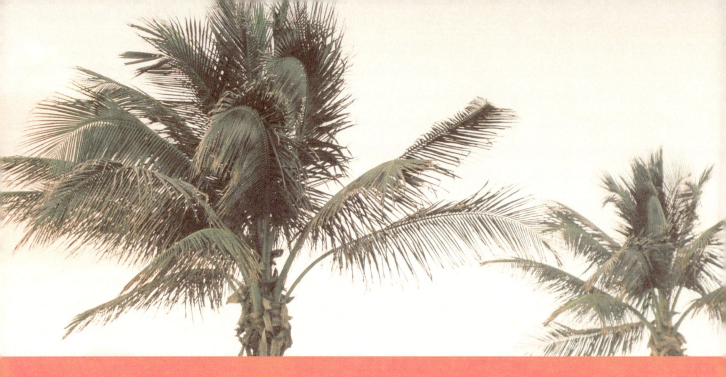

Table of Contents

Cancer is a Wanker

Cancer is a Wanker and there is simply no way around it. If this now belongs to you, I can assume you have cancer and that sucks. This journal is not going to help you fight cancer, you are going to have to do that on your own, but hopefully this journal will at least help you keep a firm hold on your sanity while you take a break from life to punch cancer in the throat. Fill this out and take pictures of the pages and send it to your people when you need them to pick up a prescription or arrange a ride home from treatment. You will be busy and you will feel like crap, let your friends help. Not the annoying ones...tell them you have it covered because people with cancer do not have to smile and deal with their annoying friends.

ALL THE DOCTORS

Find Doctors you like. Find Doctors you trust. Let the researching and the treatment analysis up to the ones that made doing that "their thing" because they are better at it than you will ever be. Find someone you trust and then trust them. Find the good ones, they will make this tolerable, they will save your life. I tend to like an ego scale of 7-8.5, I like for them to be sure of themselves but not quite a pompous asshat.

NAME:
SPECIALTY/OFFICE:
PHONE:
ADDRESS:

_____

EGO SCALE:
_____
1 2 3 4 5 6 7 8 9 10
ANNOYING / AMAZING SCALE: (CIRCLE ONE)
1 2 3 4 5 6 7 8 9 10
INTERESTING TIDBITS ABOUT THEM

_____

_____

NAME:
SPECIALTY/OFFICE:
PHONE:
ADDRESS:

_____

_____

EGO SCALE:
1 2 3 4 5 6 7 8 9 10
ANNOYING / AMAZING SCALE: (CIRCLE ONE)
1 2 3 4 5 6 7 8 9 10
INTERESTING TIDBITS ABOUT THEM

_____

_____

NAME:
SPECIALTY/OFFICE:
PHONE:
ADDRESS:

_____

_____

EGO SCALE:
1 2 3 4 5 6 7 8 9 10
ANNOYING / AMAZING SCALE: (CIRCLE ONE)
1 2 3 4 5 6 7 8 9 10
INTERESTING TIDBITS ABOUT THEM

_____

_____

NAME:
SPECIALTY/OFFICE:
PHONE:
ADDRESS:

_____

_____

EGO SCALE:
1 2 3 4 5 6 7 8 9 10
ANNOYING / AMAZING SCALE: (CIRCLE ONE)
1 2 3 4 5 6 7 8 9 10
INTERESTING TIDBITS ABOUT THEM

_____

_____

ALL THE DOCTORS

Find Doctors you like. Find Doctors you trust. Let the researching and the treatment analysis up to the ones that made doing that "their thing" because they are better at it than you will ever be. Find someone you trust and then trust them. Find the good ones, they will make this tolerable, they will save your life. I tend to like an ego scale of 7-8.5, I like for them to be sure of themselves but not quite a pompous asshat.

NAME:
SPECIALTY/OFFICE:
PHONE:
ADDRESS:

_____
EGO SCALE:
_____
1 2 3 4 5 6 7 8 9 10
ANNOYING / AMAZING SCALE: (CIRCLE ONE)
1 2 3 4 5 6 7 8 9 10
INTERESTING TIDBITS ABOUT THEM

_____
_____

NAME:
SPECIALTY/OFFICE:
PHONE:
ADDRESS:

_____
EGO SCALE:
1 2 3 4 5 6 7 8 9 10
ANNOYING / AMAZING SCALE: (CIRCLE ONE)
1 2 3 4 5 6 7 8 9 10
INTERESTING TIDBITS ABOUT THEM

_____
_____

NAME:
SPECIALTY/OFFICE:
PHONE:
ADDRESS:

_____
_____
EGO SCALE:
1 2 3 4 5 6 7 8 9 10
ANNOYING / AMAZING SCALE: (CIRCLE ONE)
1 2 3 4 5 6 7 8 9 10
INTERESTING TIDBITS ABOUT THEM

_____
_____

NAME:
SPECIALTY/OFFICE:
PHONE:
ADDRESS:

_____
_____
EGO SCALE:
1 2 3 4 5 6 7 8 9 10
ANNOYING / AMAZING SCALE: (CIRCLE ONE)
1 2 3 4 5 6 7 8 9 10
INTERESTING TIDBITS ABOUT THEM

_____
_____

PROCEDURE TRACKER

Procedure:
WTH is this doing:

_____

SIDE EFFECTS TO EXPECT

_____

ACTUAL SIDE EFFECTS

_____

RECOVERY:

_____

WHEN TO CALL THE DOC:

_____

Procedure:
WTH is this doing:

_____

SIDE EFFECTS TO EXPECT

_____

ACTUAL SIDE EFFECTS

_____

RECOVERY:

_____

WHEN TO CALL THE DOC:

_____

Procedure:
WTH is this doing:

_____

SIDE EFFECTS TO EXPECT

_____

ACTUAL SIDE EFFECTS

_____

RECOVERY:

_____

WHEN TO CALL THE DOC:

_____

Procedure:
WTH is this doing:

_____

SIDE EFFECTS TO EXPECT

_____

ACTUAL SIDE EFFECTS

_____

RECOVERY:

_____

WHEN TO CALL THE DOC:

_____

Procedure:
WTH is this doing:

_____

SIDE EFFECTS TO EXPECT

_____

ACTUAL SIDE EFFECTS

_____

RECOVERY:

_____

WHEN TO CALL THE DOC:

_____

Procedure:
WTH is this doing:

_____

SIDE EFFECTS TO EXPECT

_____

ACTUAL SIDE EFFECTS

_____

RECOVERY:

_____

WHEN TO CALL THE DOC:

_____

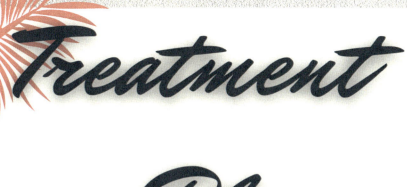

Treatment Plan

WHAT	HOW OFTEN	WHERE
WHAT	HOW OFTEN	WHERE
WHAT	HOW OFTEN	WHERE
WHAT	HOW OFTEN	WHERE

Operation Throat Punch Cancer

Operation Throat Punch Cancer is in full effect and your calendar is about full and overflowing. Keep track of your appointments and the duration of your side effects. Time shifts when you are in treatment and begins to feel like Groundhog day. Day 1: Treatment, Day 3: Nausea, Day 4: All food tastes like dirt. Track these and any other fun side effects because when a side effect normally stops on Day 4 and is lingering into Day 7, you will want to tell your doc. So write it down, chemo brain is real.

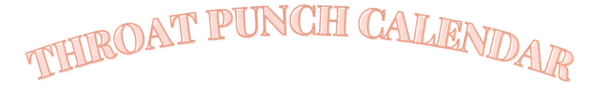

THROAT PUNCH CALENDAR

Write it down, write it all down, no sense wasting precious moments trying to wade through your drug addled, fuzzy brain trying to remember where you are supposed to be and what you are supposed to be doing.

Sunday	Monday	Tuesday	Wednesday	Thursday	Friday	Saturday

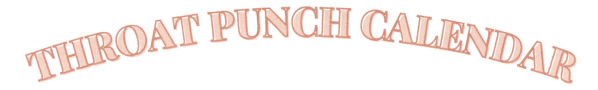

THROAT PUNCH CALENDAR

Write it down, write it all down, no sense wasting precious moments trying to wade through your drug addled, fuzzy brain trying to remember where you are supposed to be and what you are supposed to be doing.

Sunday	Monday	Tuesday	Wednesday	Thursday	Friday	Saturday

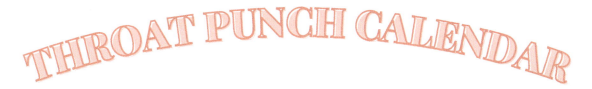

THROAT PUNCH CALENDAR

Write it down, write it all down, no sense wasting precious moments trying to wade through your drug addled, fuzzy brain trying to remember where you are supposed to be and what you are supposed to be doing.

Sunday	Monday	Tuesday	Wednesday	Thursday	Friday	Saturday

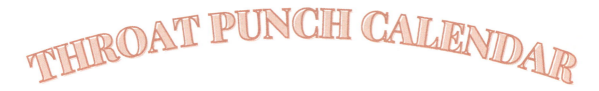

THROAT PUNCH CALENDAR

Write it down, write it all down, no sense wasting precious moments trying to wade through your drug addled, fuzzy brain trying to remember where you are supposed to be and what you are supposed to be doing.

Sunday	Monday	Tuesday	Wednesday	Thursday	Friday	Saturday

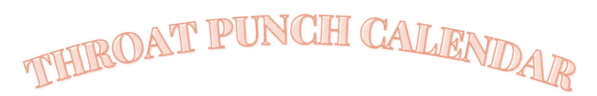

THROAT PUNCH CALENDAR

Write it down, write it all down, no sense wasting precious moments trying to wade through your drug addled, fuzzy brain trying to remember where you are supposed to be and what you are supposed to be doing.

Sunday	Monday	Tuesday	Wednesday	Thursday	Friday	Saturday

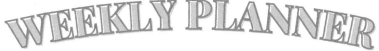

WEEKLY PLANNER

Write that Sh*t down, Chemo Brain is real.
Also, record your side effects! Side effects build up, track them and tell your Doc
when a side effect that was supposed to start chilling out on Tuesday is still
sticking around on Friday night.

Dates: _____   Treatment Week # _____

Monday:
_____
_____
MOOD:

Tuesday:
_____
_____
MOOD:

Wednesday:
_____
_____
MOOD:

Thursday:
_____
_____
MOOD:

Friday:
_____
_____
MOOD:

Saturday:
_____
_____
MOOD:

Sunday:
_____
_____
MOOD:

Well Damn, that's new:
_____
_____
SIDE EFFECT:

Side Effect Tracker
If it's annoying, if it lasts longer
than expected, write it down.

Type: _____
Duration: _____

Type: _____
Duration: _____

Type: _____
Duration: _____

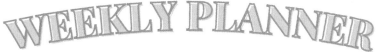

WEEKLY PLANNER

Write that Sh*t down, Chemo Brain is real.
Also, record your side effects! Side effects build up, track them and tell your Doc
when a side effect that was supposed to start chilling out on Tuesday is still
sticking around on Friday night.

Dates: Treatment Week #

Monday:
_____
_____
MOOD:

Tuesday:
_____
_____
MOOD:

Wednesday:
_____
_____
MOOD:

Thursday:
_____
_____
MOOD:

Friday:
_____
_____
MOOD:

Saturday:
_____
_____
MOOD:

Sunday:
_____
_____
MOOD:

Well Damn, that's new:
_____
_____
SIDE EFFECT:

Side Effect Tracker
If it's annoying, if it lasts longer
than expected, write it down.

Type:
_____
Duration:
_____
Type:
_____
Duration:
_____
Type:
_____
Duration:
_____

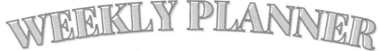
WEEKLY PLANNER

Write that Sh*t down, Chemo Brain is real.
Also, record your side effects! Side effects build up, track them and tell your Doc
when a side effect that was supposed to start chilling out on Tuesday is still
sticking around on Friday night.

Dates: _____   Treatment Week #

Monday:
_____
_____
MOOD:

Tuesday:
_____
_____
MOOD:

Wednesday:
_____
_____
MOOD:

Thursday:
_____
_____
MOOD:

Friday:
_____
_____
MOOD:

Saturday:
_____
_____
MOOD:

Sunday:
_____
_____
MOOD:

Well Damn, that's new:
_____
_____
SIDE EFFECT:

Side Effect Tracker
If it's annoying, if it lasts longer
than expected, write it down.

Type: _____
Duration: _____

Type: _____
Duration: _____

Type: _____
Duration: _____

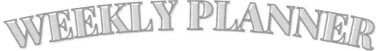

WEEKLY PLANNER

Write that Sh*t down, Chemo Brain is real.
Also, record your side effects! Side effects build up, track them and tell your Doc
when a side effect that was supposed to start chilling out on Tuesday is still
sticking around on Friday night.

Dates: Treatment Week #

Monday:
_____
_____
MOOD:

Tuesday:
_____
_____
MOOD:

Wednesday:
_____
_____
MOOD:

Thursday:
_____
_____
MOOD:

Friday:
_____
_____
MOOD:

Saturday:
_____
_____
MOOD:

Sunday:
_____
_____
MOOD:

Well Damn, that's new:
_____
_____
SIDE EFFECT:

Side Effect Tracker
If it's annoying, if it lasts longer
than expected, write it down.

Type:
_____
Duration:
_____

Type:
_____
Duration:
_____

Type:
_____
Duration:
_____

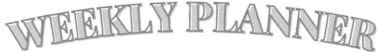

WEEKLY PLANNER

Write that Sh*t down, Chemo Brain is real.
Also, record your side effects! Side effects build up, track them and tell your Doc
when a side effect that was supposed to start chilling out on Tuesday is still
sticking around on Friday night.

Dates: _____   Treatment Week #

Monday:
_____
_____
MOOD:

Tuesday:
_____
_____
MOOD:

Wednesday:
_____
_____
MOOD:

Thursday:
_____
_____
MOOD:

Friday:
_____
_____
MOOD:

Saturday:
_____
_____
MOOD:

Sunday:
_____
_____
MOOD:

Well Damn, that's new:
_____
_____
SIDE EFFECT:

Side Effect Tracker
If it's annoying, if it lasts longer
than expected, write it down.

Type:
_____
Duration:
_____

Type:
_____
Duration:
_____

Type:
_____
Duration:
_____

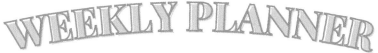

WEEKLY PLANNER

Write that Sh*t down, Chemo Brain is real.
Also, record your side effects! Side effects build up, track them and tell your Doc
when a side effect that was supposed to start chilling out on Tuesday is still
sticking around on Friday night.

Dates: _____   Treatment Week #

Monday:
_____
_____
MOOD:

Tuesday:
_____
_____
MOOD:

Wednesday:
_____
_____
MOOD:

Thursday:
_____
_____
MOOD:

Friday:
_____
_____
MOOD:

Saturday:
_____
_____
MOOD:

Sunday:
_____
_____
MOOD:

Well Damn, that's new:
_____
_____
SIDE EFFECT:

Side Effect Tracker
If it's annoying, if it lasts longer
than expected, write it down.

Type: _____
Duration: _____

Type: _____
Duration: _____

Type: _____
Duration: _____

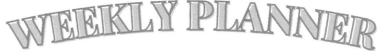

WEEKLY PLANNER

Write that Sh*t down, Chemo Brain is real.
Also, record your side effects! Side effects build up, track them and tell your Doc
when a side effect that was supposed to start chilling out on Tuesday is still
sticking around on Friday night.

Dates: _____   Treatment Week #

Monday:
_____
_____
MOOD:

Tuesday:
_____
_____
MOOD:

Wednesday:
_____
_____
MOOD:

Thursday:
_____
_____
MOOD:

Friday:
_____
_____
MOOD:

Saturday:
_____
_____
MOOD:

Sunday:
_____
_____
MOOD:

Well Damn, that's new:
_____
_____
SIDE EFFECT:

Side Effect Tracker
If it's annoying, if it lasts longer
than expected, write it down.

Type:
_____
Duration:

Type:
_____
Duration:

Type:
_____
Duration:

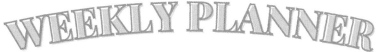
WEEKLY PLANNER

Write that Sh*t down, Chemo Brain is real.
Also, record your side effects! Side effects build up, track them and tell your Doc
when a side effect that was supposed to start chilling out on Tuesday is still
sticking around on Friday night.

Dates: Treatment Week #

Monday:
_____
_____
MOOD:

Tuesday:
_____
_____
MOOD:

Wednesday:
_____
_____
MOOD:

Thursday:
_____
_____
MOOD:

Friday:
_____
_____
MOOD:

Saturday:
_____
_____
MOOD:

Sunday:
_____
_____
MOOD:

Well Damn, that's new:
_____
_____
SIDE EFFECT:

Side Effect Tracker
If it's annoying, if it lasts longer
than expected, write it down.

Type:
_____
Duration:
_____

Type:
_____
Duration:
_____

Type:
_____
Duration:
_____

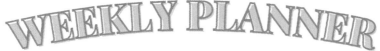

WEEKLY PLANNER

Write that Sh*t down, Chemo Brain is real.
Also, record your side effects! Side effects build up, track them and tell your Doc
when a side effect that was supposed to start chilling out on Tuesday is still
sticking around on Friday night.

Dates: _____   Treatment Week #

Monday:
_____
_____
MOOD:

Tuesday:
_____
_____
MOOD:

Wednesday:
_____
_____
MOOD:

Thursday:
_____
_____
MOOD:

Friday:
_____
_____
MOOD:

Saturday:
_____
_____
MOOD:

Sunday:
_____
_____
MOOD:

Well Damn, that's new:
_____
_____
SIDE EFFECT:

Side Effect Tracker
If it's annoying, if it lasts longer
than expected, write it down.

Type:
_____
Duration:
_____
Type:
_____
Duration:
_____
Type:
_____
Duration:
_____

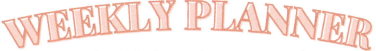
WEEKLY PLANNER

Write that Sh*t down, Chemo Brain is real.
Also, record your side effects! Side effects build up, track them and tell your Doc
when a side effect that was supposed to start chilling out on Tuesday is still
sticking around on Friday night.

Dates: _____   Treatment Week # _____

Monday:
_____
_____
MOOD:

Tuesday:
_____
_____
MOOD:

Wednesday:
_____
_____
MOOD:

Thursday:
_____
_____
MOOD:

Friday:
_____
_____
MOOD:

Saturday:
_____
_____
MOOD:

Sunday:
_____
_____
MOOD:

Well Damn, that's new:
_____
_____
SIDE EFFECT:

Side Effect Tracker
If it's annoying, if it lasts longer
than expected, write it down.

Type:
_____
Duration:
_____
Type:
_____
Duration:
_____
Type:
_____
Duration:
_____

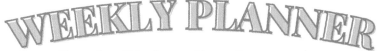

WEEKLY PLANNER

Write that Sh*t down, Chemo Brain is real.
Also, record your side effects! Side effects build up, track them and tell your Doc
when a side effect that was supposed to start chilling out on Tuesday is still
sticking around on Friday night.

Dates: _____   Treatment Week # _____

Monday:
_____
_____
MOOD:

Tuesday:
_____
_____
MOOD:

Wednesday:
_____
_____
MOOD:

Thursday:
_____
_____
MOOD:

Friday:
_____
_____
MOOD:

Saturday:
_____
_____
MOOD:

Sunday:
_____
_____
MOOD:

Well Damn, that's new:
_____
_____
SIDE EFFECT:

Side Effect Tracker
If it's annoying, if it lasts longer
than expected, write it down.

Type:
_____
Duration:
_____
Type:
_____
Duration:
_____
Type:
_____
Duration:
_____

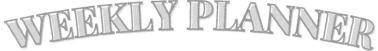

WEEKLY PLANNER

Write that Sh*t down, Chemo Brain is real.
Also, record your side effects! Side effects build up, track them and tell your Doc
when a side effect that was supposed to start chilling out on Tuesday is still
sticking around on Friday night.

Dates: _____   Treatment Week #

Monday:
_____
_____
MOOD:

Tuesday:
_____
_____
MOOD:

Wednesday:
_____
_____
MOOD:

Thursday:
_____
_____
MOOD:

Friday:
_____
_____
MOOD:

Saturday:
_____
_____
MOOD:

Sunday:
_____
_____
MOOD:

Well Damn, that's new:
_____
_____
SIDE EFFECT:

Side Effect Tracker
If it's annoying, if it lasts longer
than expected, write it down.

Type:
_____
Duration:
_____

Type:
_____
Duration:
_____

Type:
_____
Duration:
_____

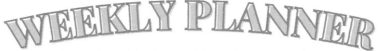

WEEKLY PLANNER

Write that Sh*t down, Chemo Brain is real.
Also, record your side effects! Side effects build up, track them and tell your Doc
when a side effect that was supposed to start chilling out on Tuesday is still
sticking around on Friday night.

Dates: _____   Treatment Week # _____

Monday:
_____
_____
MOOD:

Tuesday:
_____
_____
MOOD:

Wednesday:
_____
_____
MOOD:

Thursday:
_____
_____
MOOD:

Friday:
_____
_____
MOOD:

Saturday:
_____
_____
MOOD:

Sunday:
_____
_____
MOOD:

Well Damn, that's new:
_____
_____
SIDE EFFECT:

Side Effect Tracker
If it's annoying, if it lasts longer
than expected, write it down.

Type:
_____
Duration:
_____

Type:
_____
Duration:
_____

Type:
_____
Duration:
_____

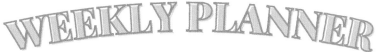

WEEKLY PLANNER

Write that Sh*t down, Chemo Brain is real.
Also, record your side effects! Side effects build up, track them and tell your Doc
when a side effect that was supposed to start chilling out on Tuesday is still
sticking around on Friday night.

Dates: _____   Treatment Week #

Monday:
_____
_____
MOOD:

Tuesday:
_____
_____
MOOD:

Wednesday:
_____
_____
MOOD:

Thursday:
_____
_____
MOOD:

Friday:
_____
_____
MOOD:

Saturday:
_____
_____
MOOD:

Sunday:
_____
_____
MOOD:

Well Damn, that's new:
_____
_____
SIDE EFFECT:

Side Effect Tracker
If it's annoying, if it lasts longer
than expected, write it down.

Type:
_____
Duration:
_____

Type:
_____
Duration:
_____

Type:
_____
Duration:
_____

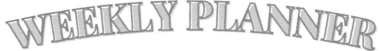

WEEKLY PLANNER

Write that Sh*t down, Chemo Brain is real.
Also, record your side effects! Side effects build up, track them and tell your Doc
when a side effect that was supposed to start chilling out on Tuesday is still
sticking around on Friday night.

Dates: _____   Treatment Week # _____

Monday:
_____
_____
MOOD:

Tuesday:
_____
_____
MOOD:

Wednesday:
_____
_____
MOOD:

Thursday:
_____
_____
MOOD:

Friday:
_____
_____
MOOD:

Saturday:
_____
_____
MOOD:

Sunday:
_____
_____
MOOD:

Well Damn, that's new:
_____
_____
SIDE EFFECT:

Side Effect Tracker
If it's annoying, if it lasts longer
than expected, write it down.

Type:
_____
Duration:
_____
Type:
_____
Duration:
_____
Type:
_____
Duration:
_____

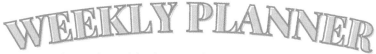

WEEKLY PLANNER

Write that Sh*t down, Chemo Brain is real.
Also, record your side effects! Side effects build up, track them and tell your Doc
when a side effect that was supposed to start chilling out on Tuesday is still
sticking around on Friday night.

Dates: _____   Treatment Week #

Monday:
_____
_____
MOOD:

Tuesday:
_____
_____
MOOD:

Wednesday:
_____
_____
MOOD:

Thursday:
_____
_____
MOOD:

Friday:
_____
_____
MOOD:

Saturday:
_____
_____
MOOD:

Sunday:
_____
_____
MOOD:

Well Damn, that's new:
_____
_____
SIDE EFFECT:

Side Effect Tracker
If it's annoying, if it lasts longer
than expected, write it down.

Type:
_____
Duration:
_____

Type:
_____
Duration:
_____

Type:
_____
Duration:
_____

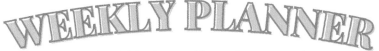

WEEKLY PLANNER

Write that Sh*t down, Chemo Brain is real.
Also, record your side effects! Side effects build up, track them and tell your Doc
when a side effect that was supposed to start chilling out on Tuesday is still
sticking around on Friday night.

Dates: _____   Treatment Week # _____

Monday:
_____
_____
MOOD:

Tuesday:
_____
_____
MOOD:

Wednesday:
_____
_____
MOOD:

Thursday:
_____
_____
MOOD:

Friday:
_____
_____
MOOD:

Saturday:
_____
_____
MOOD:

Sunday:
_____
_____
MOOD:

Well Damn, that's new:
_____
_____
SIDE EFFECT:

Side Effect Tracker
If it's annoying, if it lasts longer
than expected, write it down.

Type:
_____
Duration:
_____
Type:
_____
Duration:
_____
Type:
_____
Duration:
_____

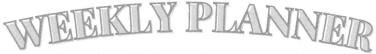

WEEKLY PLANNER

Write that Sh*t down, Chemo Brain is real.
Also, record your side effects! Side effects build up, track them and tell your Doc
when a side effect that was supposed to start chilling out on Tuesday is still
sticking around on Friday night.

Dates: _____   Treatment Week # _____

Monday:
_____
_____
MOOD:

Tuesday:
_____
_____
MOOD:

Wednesday:
_____
_____
MOOD:

Thursday:
_____
_____
MOOD:

Friday:
_____
_____
MOOD:

Saturday:
_____
_____
MOOD:

Sunday:
_____
_____
MOOD:

Well Damn, that's new:
_____
_____
SIDE EFFECT:

Side Effect Tracker
If it's annoying, if it lasts longer
than expected, write it down.

Type:
_____
Duration:
_____

Type:
_____
Duration:
_____

Type:
_____
Duration:
_____

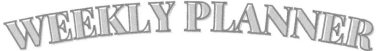

WEEKLY PLANNER

Write that Sh*t down, Chemo Brain is real.
Also, record your side effects! Side effects build up, track them and tell your Doc
when a side effect that was supposed to start chilling out on Tuesday is still
sticking around on Friday night.

Dates: _____   Treatment Week # _____

Monday:
_____
_____
MOOD:

Tuesday:
_____
_____
MOOD:

Wednesday:
_____
_____
MOOD:

Thursday:
_____
_____
MOOD:

Friday:
_____
_____
MOOD:

Saturday:
_____
_____
MOOD:

Sunday:
_____
_____
MOOD:

Well Damn, that's new:
_____
_____
SIDE EFFECT:

Side Effect Tracker
If it's annoying, if it lasts longer
than expected, write it down.

Type:
_____
Duration:
_____
Type:
_____
Duration:
_____
Type:
_____
Duration:
_____

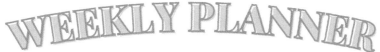

WEEKLY PLANNER

Write that Sh*t down, Chemo Brain is real.
Also, record your side effects! Side effects build up, track them and tell your Doc
when a side effect that was supposed to start chilling out on Tuesday is still
sticking around on Friday night.

Dates: _____   Treatment Week # _____

Monday:
_____
_____
MOOD:

Tuesday:
_____
_____
MOOD:

Wednesday:
_____
_____
MOOD:

Thursday:
_____
_____
MOOD:

Friday:
_____
_____
MOOD:

Saturday:
_____
_____
MOOD:

Sunday:
_____
_____
MOOD:

Well Damn, that's new:
_____
_____
SIDE EFFECT:

Side Effect Tracker
If it's annoying, if it lasts longer
than expected, write it down.

Type:
_____
Duration:
_____

Type:
_____
Duration:
_____

Type:
_____
Duration:
_____

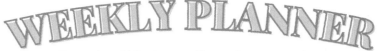

WEEKLY PLANNER

Write that Sh*t down, Chemo Brain is real.
Also, record your side effects! Side effects build up, track them and tell your Doc
when a side effect that was supposed to start chilling out on Tuesday is still
sticking around on Friday night.

Dates: _____   Treatment Week #

Monday:
_____
_____
MOOD:

Tuesday:
_____
_____
MOOD:

Wednesday:
_____
_____
MOOD:

Thursday:
_____
_____
MOOD:

Friday:
_____
_____
MOOD:

Saturday:
_____
_____
MOOD:

Sunday:
_____
_____
MOOD:

Well Damn, that's new:
_____
_____
SIDE EFFECT:

Side Effect Tracker
If it's annoying, if it lasts longer
than expected, write it down.

Type:
_____
Duration:
_____

Type:
_____
Duration:
_____

Type:
_____
Duration:
_____

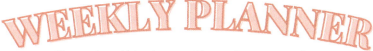

WEEKLY PLANNER

Write that Sh*t down, Chemo Brain is real.
Also, record your side effects! Side effects build up, track them and tell your Doc
when a side effect that was supposed to start chilling out on Tuesday is still
sticking around on Friday night.

Dates: _____   Treatment Week # _____

Monday:
_____
_____
MOOD:

Tuesday:
_____
_____
MOOD:

Wednesday:
_____
_____
MOOD:

Thursday:
_____
_____
MOOD:

Friday:
_____
_____
MOOD:

Saturday:
_____
_____
MOOD:

Sunday:
_____
_____
MOOD:

Well Damn, that's new:
_____
_____
SIDE EFFECT:

Side Effect Tracker
If it's annoying, if it lasts longer
than expected, write it down.

Type:
_____
Duration:
_____

Type:
_____
Duration:
_____

Type:
_____
Duration:
_____

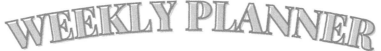

WEEKLY PLANNER

Write that Sh*t down, Chemo Brain is real.
Also, record your side effects! Side effects build up, track them and tell your Doc
when a side effect that was supposed to start chilling out on Tuesday is still
sticking around on Friday night.

Dates: _____   Treatment Week #

Monday:
_____
_____
MOOD:

Tuesday:
_____
_____
MOOD:

Wednesday:
_____
_____
MOOD:

Thursday:
_____
_____
MOOD:

Friday:
_____
_____
MOOD:

Saturday:
_____
_____
MOOD:

Sunday:
_____
_____
MOOD:

Well Damn, that's new:
_____
_____
SIDE EFFECT:

Side Effect Tracker
If it's annoying, if it lasts longer
than expected, write it down.

Type:
_____
Duration:
_____

Type:
_____
Duration:
_____

Type:
_____
Duration:
_____

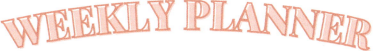

WEEKLY PLANNER

Write that Sh*t down, Chemo Brain is real.
Also, record your side effects! Side effects build up, track them and tell your Doc
when a side effect that was supposed to start chilling out on Tuesday is still
sticking around on Friday night.

Dates: _____   Treatment Week # _____

Monday:
_____
_____
MOOD:

Tuesday:
_____
_____
MOOD:

Wednesday:
_____
_____
MOOD:

Thursday:
_____
_____
MOOD:

Friday:
_____
_____
MOOD:

Saturday:
_____
_____
MOOD:

Sunday:
_____
_____
MOOD:

Well Damn, that's new:
_____
_____
SIDE EFFECT:

Side Effect Tracker
If it's annoying, if it lasts longer
than expected, write it down.

Type:
_____
Duration: _____

Type:
_____
Duration: _____

Type:
_____
Duration: _____

MY NOTES

MY NOTES

MY NOTES

MY NOTES

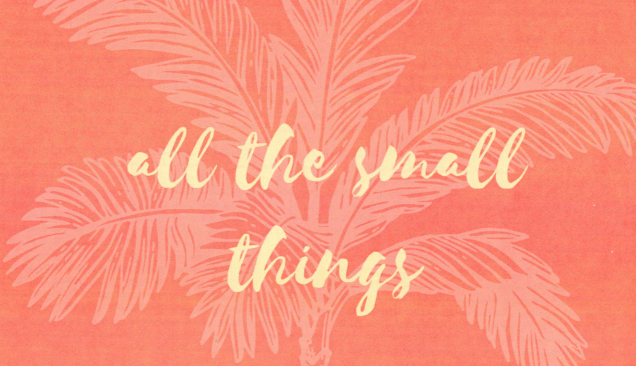

all the small things

Friends, Chemo Brain is real! Forget walking into the kitchen and forgetting what you walked in for, there will be times you are in the middle of a conversation and suddenly realize you have no idea what you are talking about. Do yourself a favor and buy a few of those beeping locators for your wallet and your keys and for the love of all things holy, write things down, because trust me...you will forget.

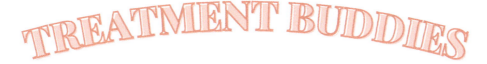

TREATMENT BUDDIES

These are the people that will not tell you to eat healthier if you ask for skittles for lunch. They are the people that will hold your hair back and not say a word if you throw up on their shoes after treatment. These are the people that will hold your hand and scream F*** into the wind before you walk into treatment, just because.

Name   *Notes*

Email

Address

Phone

•••

Name   *Notes*

Email

Address

Phone

•••

Name   *Notes*

Email

Address

Phone

•••

Name   *Notes*

Email

Address

Phone

•••

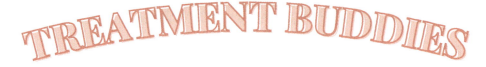

TREATMENT BUDDIES

These are the people that will not tell you to eat healthier if you ask for skittles for lunch. They are the people that will hold your hair back and not say a word if you throw up on their shoes after treatment. These are the people that will hold your hand and scream F*** into the wind before you walk into treatment, just because.

Name   *Notes*

Email

Address

Phone

- -

Name   *Notes*

Email

Address

Phone

- -

Name   *Notes*

Email

Address

Phone

- -

Name   *Notes*

Email

Address

Phone

- -

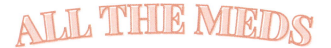

ALL THE MEDS

Buckle up, because the medications can be a doozy, most will have side effects, some will be better than others. Some you will still be cursing a decade from now. Write them down and know when you have to suck it up and when you have to call the doc!

NAME:
DOSE:
WTH IS THIS FOR:
SIDE EFFECTS:
WHEN TO CALL THE DOC:
_____
_____
WHEN TO SUCK IT UP
_____
_____

NAME:
DOSE:
WTH IS THIS FOR:
SIDE EFFECTS:
WHEN TO CALL THE DOC:
_____
_____
WHEN TO SUCK IT UP
_____
_____

NAME:
DOSE:
WTH IS THIS FOR:
SIDE EFFECTS:
WHEN TO CALL THE DOC:
_____
_____
WHEN TO SUCK IT UP
_____
_____

NAME:
DOSE:
WTH IS THIS FOR:
SIDE EFFECTS:
WHEN TO CALL THE DOC:
_____
_____
WHEN TO SUCK IT UP
_____
_____

NAME:
DOSE:
WTH IS THIS FOR:
SIDE EFFECTS:
WHEN TO CALL THE DOC:
_____
_____
WHEN TO SUCK IT UP
_____
_____

NAME:
DOSE:
WTH IS THIS FOR:
SIDE EFFECTS:
WHEN TO CALL THE DOC:
_____
_____
WHEN TO SUCK IT UP
_____
_____

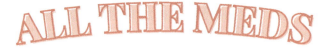

ALL THE MEDS

Buckle up, because the medications can be a doozy, most will have side effects, some will be better than others. Some you will still be cursing a decade from now. Write them down and know when you have to suck it up and when you have to call the doc!

NAME:
DOSE:
WTH IS THIS FOR:
SIDE EFFECTS:
WHEN TO CALL THE DOC:
_____
_____
WHEN TO SUCK IT UP
_____
_____

NAME:
DOSE:
WTH IS THIS FOR:
SIDE EFFECTS:
WHEN TO CALL THE DOC:
_____
_____
WHEN TO SUCK IT UP
_____
_____

NAME:
DOSE:
WTH IS THIS FOR:
SIDE EFFECTS:
WHEN TO CALL THE DOC:
_____
_____
WHEN TO SUCK IT UP
_____
_____

NAME:
DOSE:
WTH IS THIS FOR:
SIDE EFFECTS:
WHEN TO CALL THE DOC:
_____
_____
WHEN TO SUCK IT UP
_____
_____

NAME:
DOSE:
WTH IS THIS FOR:
SIDE EFFECTS:
WHEN TO CALL THE DOC:
_____
_____
WHEN TO SUCK IT UP
_____
_____

NAME:
DOSE:
WTH IS THIS FOR:
SIDE EFFECTS:
WHEN TO CALL THE DOC:
_____
_____
WHEN TO SUCK IT UP
_____
_____

ALL THE NURSES

Nurses make the world go round! They will hold your hair back and rub your back if you are sick, they will advocate and go to bat for you and you will want to remember them so you can send them chocolate on Nurses day. Nurses will save your life! Nurses are human so there are amazing and not so amazing ones but you will look back and want to remember their names and whether they prefer tea or skinny vanilla lattes.

NAME:
OFFICE:
ANNOYING / AMAZING SCALE: (CIRCLE ONE)
1 2 3 4 5 6 7 8 9 10
INTERESTING TIDBITS ABOUT THEM
_____
_____

NAME:
OFFICE:
ANNOYING / AMAZING SCALE: (CIRCLE ONE)
1 2 3 4 5 6 7 8 9 10
INTERESTING TIDBITS ABOUT THEM
_____
_____

NAME:
OFFICE:
ANNOYING / AMAZING SCALE: (CIRCLE ONE)
1 2 3 4 5 6 7 8 9 10
INTERESTING TIDBITS ABOUT THEM
_____
_____

NAME:
OFFICE:
ANNOYING / AMAZING SCALE: (CIRCLE ONE)
1 2 3 4 5 6 7 8 9 10
INTERESTING TIDBITS ABOUT THEM
_____
_____

NAME:
OFFICE:
ANNOYING / AMAZING SCALE: (CIRCLE ONE)
1 2 3 4 5 6 7 8 9 10
INTERESTING TIDBITS ABOUT THEM
_____
_____

NAME:
OFFICE:
ANNOYING / AMAZING SCALE: (CIRCLE ONE)
1 2 3 4 5 6 7 8 9 10
INTERESTING TIDBITS ABOUT THEM
_____
_____

NAME:
OFFICE:
ANNOYING / AMAZING SCALE: (CIRCLE ONE)
1 2 3 4 5 6 7 8 9 10
INTERESTING TIDBITS ABOUT THEM
_____
_____

NAME:
OFFICE:
ANNOYING / AMAZING SCALE: (CIRCLE ONE)
1 2 3 4 5 6 7 8 9 10
INTERESTING TIDBITS ABOUT THEM
_____
_____

ALL THE NURSES

Nurses make the world go round! They will hold your hair back and rub your back if you are sick, they will advocate and go to bat for you and you will want to remember them so you can send them chocolate on Nurses day. Nurses will save your life! Nurses are human so there are amazing and not so amazing ones but you will look back and want to remember their names and whether they prefer tea or skinny vanilla lattes.

NAME:
OFFICE:
ANNOYING / AMAZING SCALE: (CIRCLE ONE)
1 2 3 4 5 6 7 8 9 10
INTERESTING TIDBITS ABOUT THEM
_____
_____

NAME:
OFFICE:
ANNOYING / AMAZING SCALE: (CIRCLE ONE)
1 2 3 4 5 6 7 8 9 10
INTERESTING TIDBITS ABOUT THEM
_____
_____

NAME:
OFFICE:
ANNOYING / AMAZING SCALE: (CIRCLE ONE)
1 2 3 4 5 6 7 8 9 10
INTERESTING TIDBITS ABOUT THEM
_____
_____

NAME:
OFFICE:
ANNOYING / AMAZING SCALE: (CIRCLE ONE)
1 2 3 4 5 6 7 8 9 10
INTERESTING TIDBITS ABOUT THEM
_____
_____

NAME:
OFFICE:
ANNOYING / AMAZING SCALE: (CIRCLE ONE)
1 2 3 4 5 6 7 8 9 10
INTERESTING TIDBITS ABOUT THEM
_____
_____

NAME:
OFFICE:
ANNOYING / AMAZING SCALE: (CIRCLE ONE)
1 2 3 4 5 6 7 8 9 10
INTERESTING TIDBITS ABOUT THEM
_____
_____

NAME:
OFFICE:
ANNOYING / AMAZING SCALE: (CIRCLE ONE)
1 2 3 4 5 6 7 8 9 10
INTERESTING TIDBITS ABOUT THEM
_____
_____

NAME:
OFFICE:
ANNOYING / AMAZING SCALE: (CIRCLE ONE)
1 2 3 4 5 6 7 8 9 10
INTERESTING TIDBITS ABOUT THEM
_____
_____

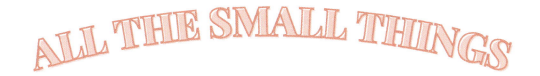

ALL THE SMALL THINGS

Just like no two snowflakes are alike, neither is anyone's cancer journey. Maybe you need to monitor your food intake, maybe you need to record the color of your poop, maybe you need to record your angry "its not fair" amazon purchase that you make late at night when you start to think about how much having cancer sucks. That goes HERE.

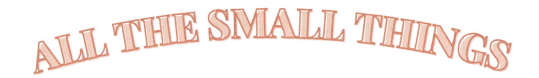

ALL THE SMALL THINGS

Retail Therapy... hell regular therapy, whatever therapy you choose, choose something that will let you escape your head a bit and then you know, keep track, because you will forget.

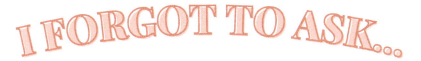

I FORGOT TO ASK...

Will this medication give me a humpback?

There will be things you forget to ask, many of them will pop into your brain at 3am...write them down...you will not remember them in the morning.

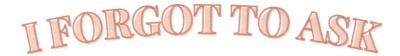

I FORGOT TO ASK

Trust me, you will need more than one page for this one!

MY NOTES

MY NOTES

MY NOTES

MY NOTES

Bloody Bucket Lists

Did Bucket list come from the idea of wanting to do things before you kicked the bucket? I don't really know but if so, that's pretty morbid for a freaking cancer journal. That being said, these bucket lists are for while you are fighting cancer with a few thrown in there for after you kick cancer in the face. You need something to look forward to and to distract you on the crappy days.

CHEMO BUCKET LIST

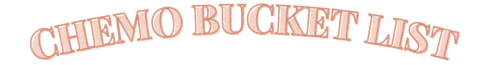

Chemotherapy...the giant time sucking, recliner rocking, sleepy inducing adventure that may save your life. It's not exactly a party, but with Wifi and the right refreshments, you may be able to finally clean out the pictures on your phone, update your Christmas card address's or binge that Netflix show that has been on your list for 4 years before the sleepies take over. Rule #1 of Cancer Fight Club is that when you are tired, your body needs sleep so I went ahead and added that to your list... don't be an dingbat and ignore that one, its in bold for a reason.

- **TAKE A FREAKING NAP**

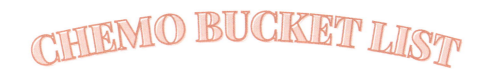

CHEMO BUCKET LIST

I added a second page for you Type A Overachievers...napping is still a requirement...even for you

_____

_____

_____

_____

_____

_____

_____

_____

- **TAKE A FREAKING NAP**

_____

BOOK BUCKET LIST

Make a list of all the books you want to read after this suckfest is over. Committing to finishing a book during cancer can be difficult due to that super annoying side effect of always falling asleep which tends to accompany most cancer treatments. Despite that, you will get a lot of book recommendations, may as well write them down.

TITLE:
WHO REFERRED THIS:
DO YOU TRUST THE RECCOMENDATION:
1 2 3 4 5 6 7 8 9 10
NOTES:
_____
_____

TITLE:
WHO REFERRED THIS:
DO YOU TRUST THE RECCOMENDATION:
1 2 3 4 5 6 7 8 9 10
NOTES:
_____
_____

TITLE:
WHO REFERRED THIS:
DO YOU TRUST THE RECCOMENDATION:
1 2 3 4 5 6 7 8 9 10
NOTES:
_____
_____

TITLE:
WHO REFERRED THIS:
DO YOU TRUST THE RECCOMENDATION:
1 2 3 4 5 6 7 8 9 10
NOTES:
_____
_____

TITLE:
WHO REFERRED THIS:
DO YOU TRUST THE RECCOMENDATION:
1 2 3 4 5 6 7 8 9 10
NOTES:
_____
_____

TITLE:
WHO REFERRED THIS:
DO YOU TRUST THE RECCOMENDATION:
1 2 3 4 5 6 7 8 9 10
NOTES:
_____
_____

BOOK BUCKET LIST

TITLE:
WHO REFERRED THIS:
DO YOU TRUST THE RECCOMENDATION:
1 2 3 4 5 6 7 8 9 10
NOTES:

_____
_____

TITLE:
WHO REFERRED THIS:
DO YOU TRUST THE RECCOMENDATION:
1 2 3 4 5 6 7 8 9 10
NOTES:

_____
_____

TITLE:
WHO REFERRED THIS:
DO YOU TRUST THE RECCOMENDATION:
1 2 3 4 5 6 7 8 9 10
NOTES:

_____
_____

TITLE:
WHO REFERRED THIS:
DO YOU TRUST THE RECCOMENDATION:
1 2 3 4 5 6 7 8 9 10
NOTES:

_____
_____

TITLE:
WHO REFERRED THIS:
DO YOU TRUST THE RECCOMENDATION:
1 2 3 4 5 6 7 8 9 10
NOTES:

_____
_____

TITLE:
WHO REFERRED THIS:
DO YOU TRUST THE RECCOMENDATION:
1 2 3 4 5 6 7 8 9 10
NOTES:

_____
_____

TITLE:
WHO REFERRED THIS:
DO YOU TRUST THE RECCOMENDATION:
1 2 3 4 5 6 7 8 9 10
NOTES:

_____
_____

TITLE:
WHO REFERRED THIS:
DO YOU TRUST THE RECCOMENDATION:
1 2 3 4 5 6 7 8 9 10
NOTES:

_____
_____

GET THE HELL OUT OF DODGE

AKA Vacations you would like to take after this sh*t is over, places you would like to see, dream big.

MY NOTES

MY NOTES

MY NOTES

MY NOTES

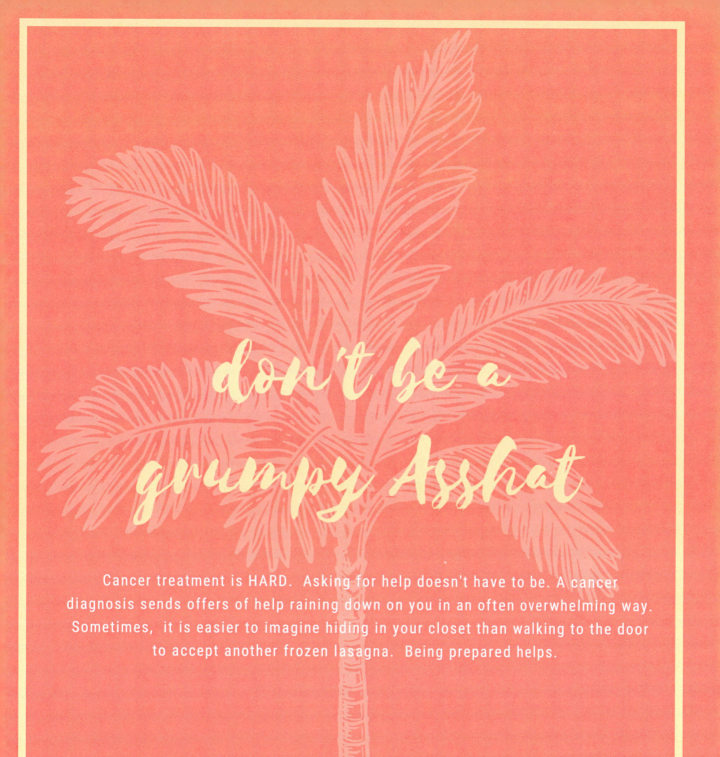

don't be a grumpy Asshat

Cancer treatment is HARD. Asking for help doesn't have to be. A cancer diagnosis sends offers of help raining down on you in an often overwhelming way. Sometimes, it is easier to imagine hiding in your closet than walking to the door to accept another frozen lasagna. Being prepared helps.

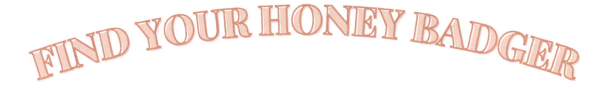

FIND YOUR HONEY BADGER

No one messes with a honey badger. Find your honey badger and put them to work. This is the person that will send out a group text intercepting your friends and family with a notification that updates come through them because you are tired, and sending the same text to 49 people every week is exhausting. This is the person that will tell people to put your dinner drop offs in a cooler on the porch because no matter how much you love them, making small talk on the porch each night is emotionally draining. Your Honey badger will be your mouth piece and they will guard you fiercely. Say Thank You!

MY HONEY BADGER

_____

_____

_____

_____

TREATS FOR MY HONEY BADGER

_____

_____

_____

CHORES I HATE

Offers of help will rain down on you, you do not have to accept them all, you do not have to accept any of them, just know that they are coming from love and a feeling of helplessness. Your people cannot fight cancer for you so they offer anything and everything to try to make it easier. If walking the dog is your mental Zen garden, then by all means walk your own damn dog. If mowing the yard sucks...boom, that's a way someone can help.

Pro Tip: Take a picture of this Page and send it to your Honey badger, they can assign these chores, while you take that damn nap!

FOODS I LOVE

There is nothing like a meal train gone wrong...it's a blessing to not have think about dinner. It's aggravating to have to take the vodka out of the freezer to make room for a 7th frozen lasagna that you are not going to eat.

_____

_____

_____

_____

_____

_____

FOOD ALLERGIES

_____

_____

_____

_____

Pro Tip: Take a picture of this Page and send it to your Honey badger, they can let everyone know your preferences, while you take that damn nap!

FOODS I HATE

If you would rather eat dirt than stuffed shells, write it down here and let your Honey Badger lovingly convey that. A food train only works if it really makes life easier by taking away the chore of making dinner.

UMM, MY FAMILY WON'T EAT THAT

Pro Tip: Take a picture of this Page and send it to your Honey badger, they can let everyone know that stuffed shells make you dry heave.

MY NOTES

MY NOTES

MY NOTES

well color me
calm

Will coloring make the stress of cancer disappear, probably not...will it distract you for a few minutes and just let you breathe...yes, it freaking will.

COLOR

Its a thing, doodling, coloring.. it lowers your blood pressure or your heart rate! Actually I don't know if it does either of those but its calming AF so if you are aggravated start filling in the lines!!

You are
kind

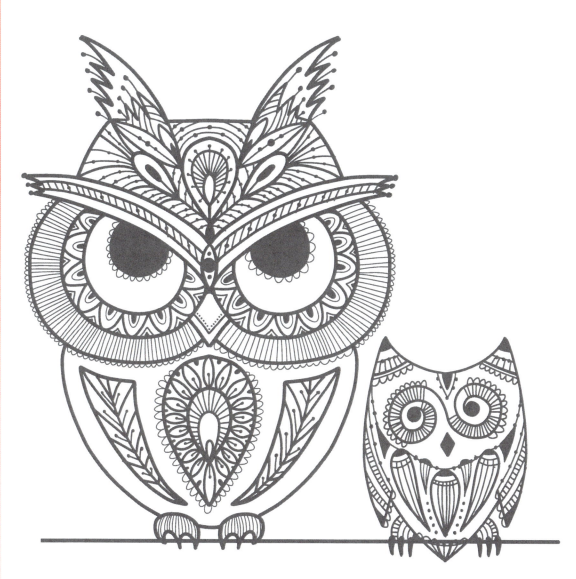

You are
loved

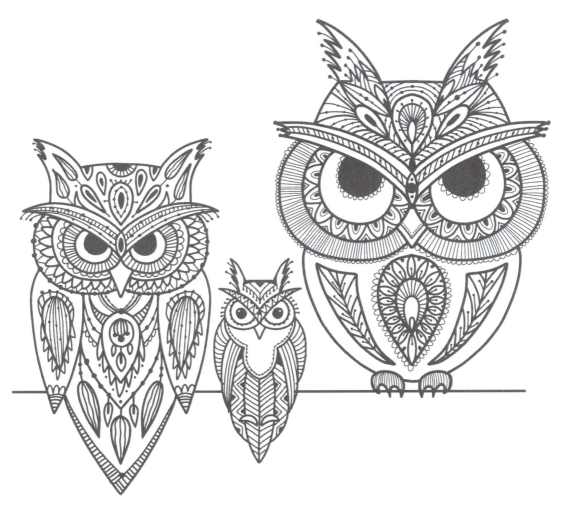

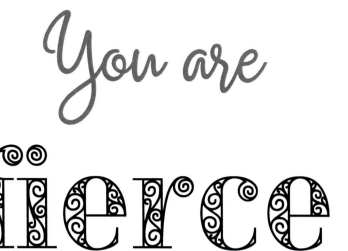

You are

fierce

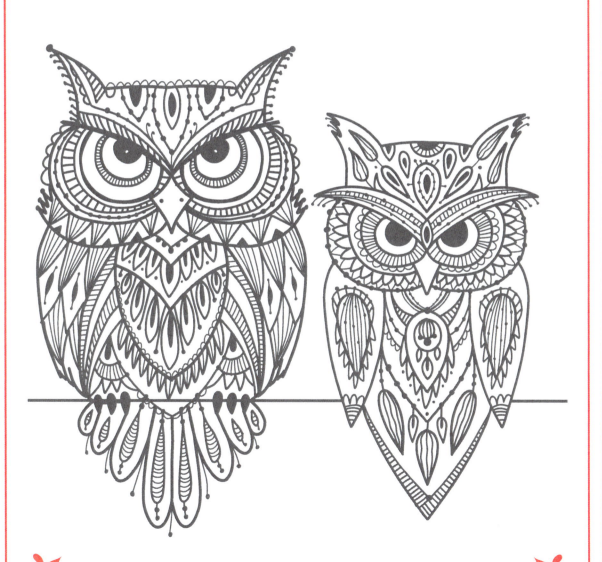

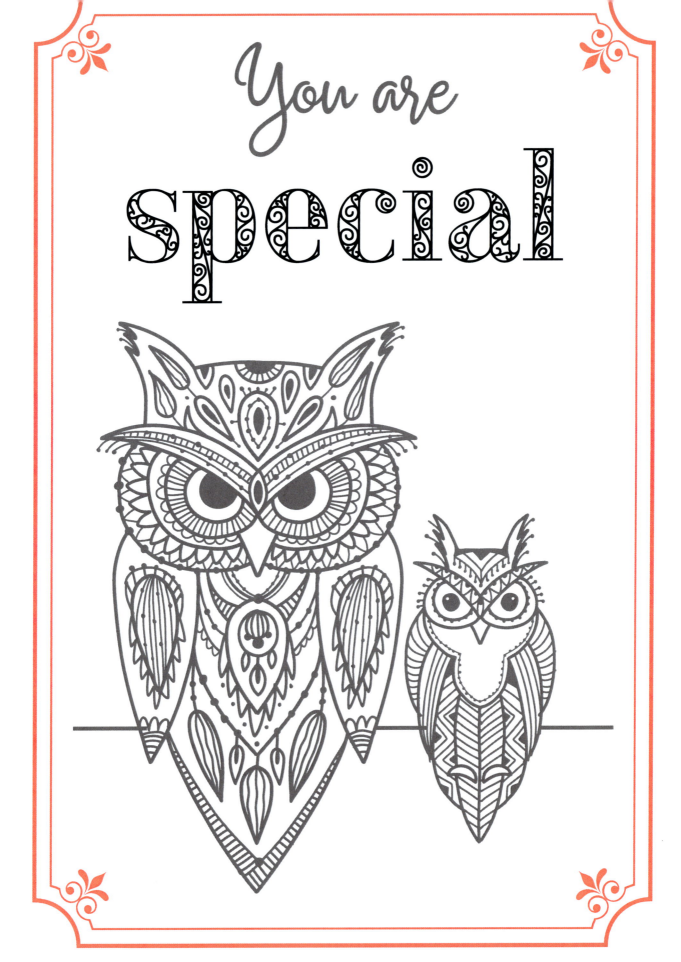

You are
enough

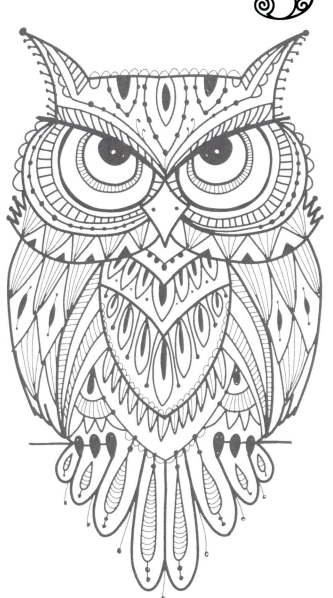

Go Home Cancer, You're Drunk

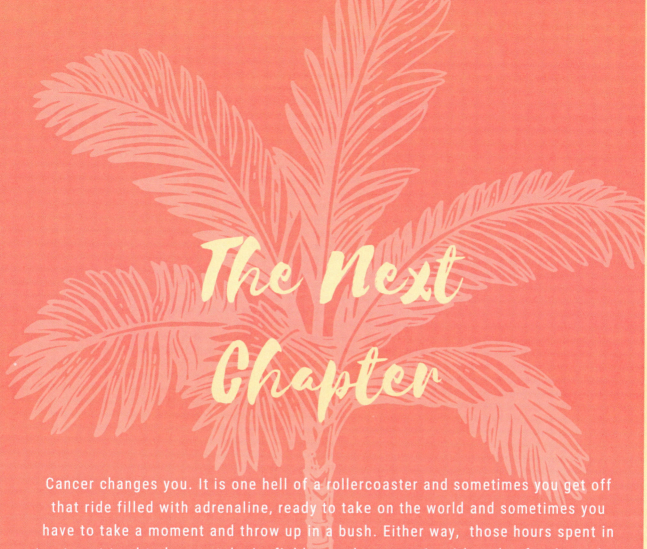

The Next Chapter

Cancer changes you. It is one hell of a rollercoaster and sometimes you get off that ride filled with adrenaline, ready to take on the world and sometimes you have to take a moment and throw up in a bush. Either way, those hours spent in treatment tend to be mental minefield, so why not go in with a plan for the end or at the very least spend some time thinking about anything but cancer.

THINGS THAT MEAN THE MOST

What are the things in life that mean the most. The traditions, the activities, the things in life that bring you the most joy. Be specific. Don't write "family", write "baking Christmas cookies with the aunties"

_____

_____

_____

_____

_____

_____

_____

_____

_____

_____

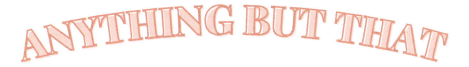

ANYTHING BUT THAT

What are the things in life that bring you NO joy. Record the things you do because you "should" and not because you want to. Write down *what* and even *who* sucks the life out of you and then think about how to walk away because YOU are important, you deserve real joy and it is freaking ok to say NO Thank you.

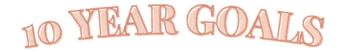

10 YEAR GOALS

If you could do anything / be anything / live anywhere...no constraints...write it down. DREAM BIG. Dream bigger than you think you should! If it's not scary or it doesn't feel impossible, it's not big enough.

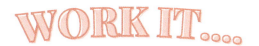

WORK IT....

Pick a goal and write down 5 things that scare the hell out of you when you think of pursuing that dream. Below it right down 1 thing you can do to overcome that fear and get closer to that goal...the things don't have to get you the whole way there...just closer!

1.
⭐

2.
⭐

3.
⭐

4.
⭐

5.
⭐

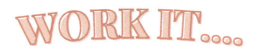

WORK IT....

Oh hell, pick another goal and do it again

1.
⭐

2.
⭐

3.
⭐

4.
⭐

5.
⭐

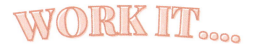

WORK IT....

Imagine someone living the life you want.
What is different about their everyday life. When do they wake up, what do they make a priority, what habits do they repeat. Write it down, below those things write down a few simple things you could do to intentionally shift your reality towards the life you want.

1.

⭐

2.

⭐

3.

⭐

4.

⭐

5.

⭐

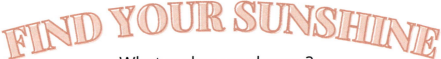

FIND YOUR SUNSHINE

What makes you happy?
Happiness isn't found, it is made. You choose happiness. You create happiness, this one is totally on you and no one else, so figure it out. What can you do to make YOUR joy a bigger priority in your next chapter. Write it down. BE SPECIFIC. Don't write "relaxing", write "eating lucky charms in the bathtub while I watch trashy TV on the Ipad" and then do it and dammit don't apologize for it!!

_____

_____

_____

_____

_____

_____

_____

_____

_____

_____

MY NOTES

MY NOTES

MY NOTES

MY NOTES

Made in the USA
Monee, IL
11 July 2022